Intermittent Fasting — Beginners Guide

The Ultimate Diet Guide for Men and Women who Want to Reset Their Metabolism, Lose Weight, Increase Energy, and Detox for a Healthier Life

Elouisa Smith

Table of Contents

A Fast Introduction

Intermittent fasting is the simplest way to lose excess weight and achieve a healthy new you. Whether you're curious, skeptical, or excited to get started, it can be confusing to know how to get started when there is so much information out! Intermittent fasting is a widely covered subject. Let me save you the frustration right now and tell you exactly what it is. Intermittent fasting is the scheduled control of burning off stored energy sources. When you fast, your body uses its stored fat as energy. That's it. We'll get into the scientific details soon; however, the basic premise is that when you eat, you store fat. When you fast, you burn fat. The longer you fast, the more fat you'll burn.

Fasting is not a new concept. In fact, it dates back to prehistoric times. Think along the lines of cave dwellers and hunter/gatherers. Prehistoric humans fasted out of necessity as food was difficult to come by or keep preserved. Whether due to scarcity of prey or bad weather, they would go for days without a proper meal, yet their bodies survived.

Moving along in time, according to Britannica (2021) in the fifth century, the physician Hippocrates saw the benefits of fasting and recommended that patients not eat or drink while ill. He supported his theory by the fact that patients would lose their appetite when experiencing certain illnesses. They recognized what the human body was telling them, perhaps they didn't understand it scientifically, but they listened to nature's recovery processes and used it as a treatment.

Within various religious beliefs and cultures, fasting was (and is still) used to pay penance or show devotion. But some see fasting as a spiritual endeavor. As I'm sure you can imagine, to fast for days or weeks at a time would take quite a bit of determination and strength of mind. If fasters become dehydrated or malnourished, they could experience delirium and hallucinations, which would then be perceived as a spiritual or religious experience. Regardless, cultures that believe in regular fasting have been found to live longer and healthier lives throughout history (Langness, 2019).

Intermittent fasting is a modern version of sustaining oneself without food but without the life-threatening risks because we have food readily available. Science has recognized the benefits of fasting, and we've adapted it to suit our needs. Whether those needs are to lose weight or prevent disease, intermittent fasting can benefit you somehow.

Fasting is a concept that scares a lot of people while others are absolutely in love with it. But we've all already been fasting all our lives! While you sleep, you're fasting. While you aren't eating, you're fasting. Think about how easy that makes it sound? Not so scary anymore. It's just a matter of prolonging that amount of time you're not eating. Fasting has become an increasingly popular way of losing weight and bettering general health for the last few years, as science continues to debunk old ways of dieting. Today, it's actually encouraged to eat red meats and healthy fats instead of cutting your diet right down to a stick of celery.

There is no diet plan, no workout plan, nor is there a restrictive way of living. It's an eating schedule, and the rules are entirely up to you! Intermittent fasting starts with skipping a meal; if you are used to skipping meals, you're already halfway there. Especially within busy lifestyles, it's easy enough to skip breakfast for a cup of coffee instead. It's easy enough to work through an entire eight-hour shift without even thinking about food if you're keeping busy. Granted, if you're not that busy, it could be difficult. But what better reason is there to get busy? Distract yourself with activities you love! You'll have enough time now that you're not cooking three times a day every day.

Read on, and you'll fall in love with fasting as well. Discover how and why it works, how easy it can be, and how easily it can fit into your lifestyle. This book should answer all your questions. It will explain the science behind fasting and how it works within the body. You'll find out just how much your health can benefit from it. I'll explain to you how you can incorporate intermittent fasting into your lifestyle and which type of fast might be best for you based on your goals. By reading this book, you'll learn just how simple and easy intermittent fasting really is.

Chapter 1: Fast Facts — The Science Behind the Craze

Everyone is getting into intermittent fasting. It's the most popular weight loss plan right now. You might call it a craze; however, it's not crazy at all. While many are already sold on the concept, many others are skeptical. They aren't sure of the safety, the difficulty, the rules, or the credibility of what others tell them. The first chapter will answer all of these questions first before we get into any dietary details.

First and foremost, we'll discuss the terminology because if you've done any research or checked any intermittent fasting forums, you probably saw a few words or acronyms and thought, "What does that mean?!" Well, I'm going to help you understand the basics. Then I'm going to discuss the craze.

Whenever a new diet plan comes along, everyone gets excited. Either they're all for it and change their entire lives for it, or they are completely against it and preach about why it isn't good for you. Then there are the skeptics; those people who brush it off and say that it's just another craze, it won't help them, nothing that sounds too good to be true is ever actually true. If you fall into the last two categories, this first chapter is for you. We'll discuss the craze of intermittent fasting and whether what people are saying is true or not. Lastly, we'll give you the actual scientific facts about fasting and explain the processes behind the concept, proving how it can help you.

The Terminology

When trying to understand intermittent fasting as a beginner, things can get confusing. It's as if everyone who is already fasting has this language they use that any newbie would struggle to keep up with! Whether it's a simple acronym or a scientific term, it's important to understand what you're reading so that you know how to apply it to your life or diet. Some terminologies and acronyms that aren't necessarily general knowledge are the follows:

IF — Intermittent Fasting

OMAD — One Meal A Day

ADF — Alternate Day Fasting

LCHF — Low-Carb High-Fat diet

BMR — Basal Metabolic Rate. The rate at which your body burns calories while you're not doing anything or while you're sleeping. Also called Resting Metabolic Rate (RMR).

AMR — Active Metabolic Rate. The rate at which your body burns calories while you're active during the day.

'Clean' eating — Eating only fresh foods, no processed or refined foods.

'Clean' fasting — Drinking only water, coffee and tea without any flavorings, sugar, or dairy added.

Ketosis — A state your body enters when it uses ketones for bodily energy instead of glucose, which assists in burning off stored fat. For example, the popular ketogenic diet involves cutting all forms of glucose (carbohydrates and starch sugar content) from your meals.

Autophagy — The process of removing damaged cell parts and repairing the body cells. It promotes growth and healing of the body.

Glucose, glycogen and glucagon — These three words can be easily confused. Glucose is the sugar in your blood, glycogen is the chain-like combination of glucose particles the body creates for storage within your liver or muscle mass, and glucagon is the hormone that lets the liver know to start turning the glycogen back into glucose for energy use. (Glucagon is the opposite hormone of insulin, which tells the liver to store glucose as glycogen.)

Knowing the above terms will make understanding how IF works much easier for you. They might feel out of context at this point, but soon you'll begin to see the relevance.

The Craze

Intermittent fasting has become extremely popular, probably because of the leniency that it gives you in not restricting what you can eat within your eating window. But it's also because of the results. Many people have had great results using IF in their lives, in terms of weight loss and improving general health and bodily energy. This only makes others want to try it even more. So, everyone jumps on the bandwagon and gives it a try. The issue comes in when people start fasting without doing their research. Many question the safety of any kind of fasting at all but the truth is that it is safe if you're monitoring yourself and eating correctly. IF doesn't work well if you counteract it with an unhealthy lifestyle. Also, don't believe everything you see online. IF is a different process for everyone, and most times, you need to figure it out for yourself. Many people are doling out advice about how to fast, and much of it isn't true. Let's debunk some myths that are all over the internet:

Myth 1: The Craze over Metabolic Rates

Some people believe that if you eat smaller portions more frequently, you can increase your metabolism and burn off calories faster. They also state that IF can slow your metabolism because you're not eating, so your body will try to preserve its calories by burning less. Not true. Your metabolic rate concerns how fast your body is burning calories, and how often you eat won't change that. Undereating will do that, so as long as you're ingesting the same number of calories during your eating window, your metabolism should stay the same (Pannell, 2018).

Myth 2: Fasting Increases Hunger

The belief that eating more frequently reduces hunger causes certain people to deduce that fasting will make you feel ravenously hungry. This is not completely true. Naturally, eating more often will keep you feeling full and therefore not hungry. But it doesn't reduce your hunger; it could be making it worse. Your body will get used to the constant intake of food, and when that stops, you'll feel hungry. However, once your body becomes accustomed to fasting, it won't expect food but instead burn off stored energy. When your body is used to using stored energy, your appetite hormones stabilize, and you don't feel as hungry.

Myth 3: You are 'Allowed' to Overindulge After a Fast

Not really true if you want to see results. IF is based on the timeframe of your meals, not the size of your meals. So as long as you eat the same number of calories as you normally would, or less, you should see results. If you end up eating more calories than you used to, you won't see results. Remember that all the time you spend fasting is time during which you aren't taking in calories. Make sure that during your eating window you don't let that time go to waste.

Myth 4: You Don't Digest Food When You Sleep

Some believe IF works because you don't digest food at night (which is why you should stop eating earlier in the evening). This is not true. Your body will digest food at any time, no matter what. The reason IF works is because you're giving your body a longer period in which it can finish digesting and burning through the energy (glucose) in your blood in order to start burning stored fat. It also gives your body time to use the energy it's burning on other processes such as cellular repair instead of constantly focusing its energies on digestion.

The last thing I'd like to point out is not so much of a myth as it is a misunderstanding. In terms of weight loss, some people use a method similar to IF, but they don't completely fast; they only restrict calories. So they may follow the same time frames, but not necessarily the same 'rule' as a complete fast. They will be more precise about measuring calories and set a goal of, say, cutting calories down to a quarter of their usual intake during that period of time. To give you an example, a person would eat normally for five days of the week but eat a significantly lower number of calories for two days. This can apply to any of the fasting schedules discussed in chapter three, but it isn't technically a fast.

The Science

The Processes That Occur When You Eat

When you eat, you are giving your body energy. The food is broken down during digestion, and the sugar content becomes glucose in your blood. This glucose is the most direct source of energy for your body to use as it's readily available in your bloodstream. Usually, when we eat, there will be more energy than our bodies can use at once, so the extra energy is stored for later use. Insulin assists in storing the excess glucose as glycogen in the liver and muscle mass. Once there is no more room for glycogen, it will turn the extra glucose into fat and store it elsewhere in the body as fat deposits. As soon as you eat again, your glucose (blood sugar) will rise again, and your body will continue to use that as its energy source while storing the excess. By not giving your body the chance to use the energy it's been given, it will only keep storing the excess as fat.

The Processes That Occur When You Don't Eat

When you stop eating, the body will first go through the process mentioned above. Glucose and insulin levels will rise, assisting the body in using and storing energy. Eventually, glucose levels in the blood will start to decrease as your body uses it for energy. Insulin will then decrease, slowing down the process of storing excess energy as the body gets ready to use its stored energy. It then uses the glycogen stored in the liver and muscle mass to produce energy. Once the levels of glycogen decrease, the body will get ready to use its stored fat. This is why fasting is the most straightforward way to lose weight because you're giving your body the chance to start using its stored fat.

The Four Bodily States

To be able to understand fasting schedules and how they differ in benefits, you need to understand the timeline of the above-mentioned processes. The body goes through four different states, each state adapting and changing processes to preserve the body and keep energy levels up.

The 'fed state' occurs during the first three to four hours after eating. The body digests the food and breaks it down to absorb the nutrients. This is when your glucose and insulin levels increase. Other hormones are affected as well that regulate your appetite. Ghrelin stimulates your appetite while leptin decreases it. After eating, leptin will rise, telling your body that you're full.

The 'early fasting state' occurs between four and 18 hours after eating. During this time, your glucose and insulin levels slowly decrease, so your body starts to make other plans for energy. First, the glycogen in your liver and muscle mass is converted back to glucose to be used for energy. This is normally when most people will decide to eat again after fasting for 18 hours. However, some continue into the next stage.

The 'fasting state' occurs between the 18th and 48th hours after eating. Your body is now looking for alternative energy sources of energy as your glycogen stores run low. Another source of energy will come from various proteins stored within your muscle mass, which are broken down into molecules called amino acids and then used as an energy source. Once your body reaches a point where there is no more glucose, it starts breaking down your stored fats. The resulting energy source molecules are called ketones. Your body is slowly entering a state of ketosis in which your body's main source of energy comes from fats instead of glucose.

The 'long-term fasting state' occurs two days after eating (48 hours and above). Sometimes known as the starvation state. However, IF should never be considered starvation because you're choosing not to eat, it's under your control. Some people choose to continue their fast after 48 hours as the body continues to break down stored fats even faster. Your insulin level continues to decrease as there is no glucose to store, while your ketone level continues to rise as it feeds your body energy from stored fat. The breakdown of amino acids (proteins) now slows down as the body preserves your muscle mass, meaning the body is even more reliant on stored fats for energy. This bodily state can be dangerous and is not recommended unless first discussed with your health practitioner.

Chapter 2: Fasting Effects — The Health Benefits

Whenever you hear about intermittent fasting, it usually has to do with weight loss; however, there are so many more benefits. We've learned now that the reason IF works so well is because it's giving your body time to catch up with processes that it normally doesn't have the time or energy to do. Sound familiar? Imagine that your boss told you that you only have to work four days a week, or three days a week. Imagine what you could do with that extra free time! Not only would you be less stressed, but you'd have time to focus on yourself and do the things you never get the time to do. Now imagine your body gets the same memo; suddenly, it doesn't need to focus solely on digesting every single thing you put into your mouth (for example, small meals frequently throughout the day), but now has the time to focus on healing itself! Your body is less stressed and can now serve you better because of it. Once your body reaches a state where it's no longer using glucose for energy but is now sourcing energy from ketone molecules, it activates a process called autophagy, and this is when the benefits start rolling in.

The Health Benefits of Fasting Explained

Weight Loss

The most obvious reason why IF can help you lose weight is that you essentially eat less. Even if you try to eat the same amount of food during your eating window as you would on a normal eating day, chances are that you'll become full and not want to eat so much. You will probably end up eating the same portion meals, just less often, and so you will unknowingly consume fewer calories because you have to cut yourself off at an earlier point than you would have before. If your goal is to lose weight, you will need to eat the correct foods during your eating window, which have fewer calories. So altogether the number of calories you're consuming should be less, as long as you're not binge eating cinnamon rolls covered in icing after you fast. Another factor in losing weight through IF is based on your insulin level. A major driving factor behind IF as a concept is that it gives your body time for your insulin level to decrease. As long as it's decreasing, the glucagon level is increasing, and stored fat is being released. It's that simple.

We have discussed the scientific processes that your body goes through the longer your fast lasts, so we know that the longer the fast, the more stored fat will be used. The longer you go without food the more your body will try to preserve your muscle mass and nutrients, which is why during the fourth bodily state, the long term fasting state, amino acids from proteins kept within muscle mass are no longer being used as an alternative energy source. This means that stored fats are the only source left to use, increasing the rate at which those fats are burned off. Simply put, the longer you fast, the more weight you're losing. This is why some people find it more beneficial to eat during their usual time frame of 12:12, according to a weight loss diet plan for a few days, and then fast for at least 36 hours up to 72 hours. This should only be done once a month and your health practitioner should be consulted if you're considering this fasting timeline.

We will discuss dietary plans in the next chapter; however, it is important to note here that the most effective way to lose weight with IF is to cut calories. When you are eating, try to eat only clean foods with as little a calorie intake as you can handle. Many people benefit from combining the ketogenic diet plan with intermittent fasting, as they complement each other and achieve the best results.

Metabolism Reset

When you've fasted for at least 18 hours, your body slowly crosses over from using glucose as its main source of energy to using ketones instead. Everyone's timeline will be different; however, ketosis will begin between 18 and 48 hours after eating. This is called the metabolic switch. You've reset the way your body creates energy. Research has found that when your body switches from using glucose as its main energy source to using ketones that are sourced from fatty acids (stored fats), it triggers a shift in your metabolism from one type of process to another, namely from fat-storing processes to taking fat from storage through the process of creating ketones. When this switch is made, various other functions are enhanced as well.

Aside from a complete reset in metabolism, intermittent fasting can help you better your metabolic rate and metabolic health. IF is known to have a stabilizing effect on various hormones in your body. Insulin is one example. It keeps your insulin levels low and therefore not storing fats. Another is the human growth hormone (HGH), which increases during a fast and promotes fat burning, as well as preserving muscle mass. When muscle mass is preserved, your metabolic rate is better because muscle tissue burns calories. Therefore, the more muscle you have, the more calories you're burning off, and the faster your metabolic rate is.

If you are concerned about keeping your metabolic rate high, sleep! When you sleep for longer periods of time, your metabolic rate is better. This is because your resting metabolic rate (RMR), or basal metabolic rate (BMR), is higher than your active metabolic rate (AMR). What better way is there to get through a difficult fasting period than sleeping through it? Sleep is, after all, the original intermittent fasting inspirer. Everyone fasts while they sleep. But if you can sleep and therefore fast for longer, your metabolic rate will be better. Another option is to incorporate meditation into your fasting periods. The stress hormone, cortisol, reduces your metabolic rate. Therefore, less stress, higher metabolic rate.

Detoxification

During the third and fourth stages of fasting states (18 hours after eating), as discussed, your body's glucose supply runs low, and it begins sourcing energy from elsewhere in the body. At that point, your insulin levels are low, meaning your glucagon levels are high. This is the hormone that tells your liver to turn any glucose it receives into energy instead of stored fat. As this happens, it triggers another process into action — autophagy. The rise in ketones supports this process as well as it supplies the body's cells with more energy. Since your body is now in a fasting state, its energy is spread to cellular and brain activity instead of digestion. Autophagy is the process of old and damaged cell parts being removed and broken down to become amino acids to be used for energy. The cells are then refurbished with new cell parts thanks to a rise in the human growth hormone (HGH).

This is how fasting can help repair and grow your body as well as how it detoxifies it. Over time, toxins from eating unhealthy processed foods, called advanced glycation end products (AGE), start to build up in your cellular tissues. If you aren't getting enough nutrients to detoxify your body, that build-up will worsen. When autophagy happens, those toxins are part of what is removed. Your cells are cleansed, and cellular repair begins. The buildup of toxins is what can cause diseases such as Alzheimer's or cancer (Gunnars, 2016). By flushing them out, you lower your risk of disease significantly. Many of the toxins that come from eating processed and refined foods are stored in the body's fat deposits as well. So, when you burn off fat, you're also burning off toxins. If I had to choose which health benefit is the best one, this would be it. Not only will IF help detox your body, but it can prolong your life and leave you a healthier human being.

Energy Increase

When your body begins to reap the benefits of fasting, you will begin to experience an increase in body energy. This won't happen immediately but will come with regular fasting and being in a regular state of ketosis. If you consider the history of humans, they used to survive with only energy from healthy fats and proteins as they had no processed foods or refined carbohydrates. Once we started creating these foods, our bodies adapted to the new levels of blood sugar and began using it as its primary source of energy.

In my mind, this proves that living off of energy produced through carbohydrates and starch sugars (glucose) is an unhealthy type of fuel, and that's why the body wants to burn it off first before anything else. Once you flip that metabolic switch and begin producing energy from fats (ketones) and proteins (amino acids), it's a healthy kind of fuel. Ketones are said to possibly produce more energy than glucose. The benefit of being in a ketogenic state is that many of your body's functions are improved. One of these functions is in fact the production of energy itself. This happens in the part of the body and brain cells called mitochondria. When your body begins autophagy and cellular repair, these mitochondria are increased and become more efficient, therefore producing more healthy energy.

A fantastic example of how IF can improve your overall energy and brain function is that of Kyle Boelte (2017), who wrote about his experience with beginning intermittent fasting. He was a fit and healthy man who exercised regularly and ate frequently throughout the day. However, he found he would still need a nap every afternoon. After a few years of various doctors' considerations and failures to diagnose him, he finally decided to give IF a try. He came to realize that his issue with tiredness (chronic lethargy) was due to his blood sugar levels spiking and dropping because of his eating patterns and workouts. He was dependent on the energy that he gained from eating carbohydrates and would need to top himself off regularly.

He began fasting by simply putting breakfast off for an hour in the morning and eating an hour earlier in the evening. He considered IF as if it were exercise. A person who doesn't exercise won't just start running marathons one day. They need to start gradually and become used to it. It will put your body through a small amount of stress each time you make a change, but this is how you'll adapt and start benefitting. He calls this "beneficial stress," similar to the type of stress your muscles and heart endure during exercise. Eventually, he became used to a 16:8 type fasting regime, and no longer needs afternoon naps. He didn't find it restrictive at all and, in fact, points out that you don't need to be absolutely strict about the eating schedule. If you need to eat earlier because you're tired or working out, do so. And if you want to go for a late dinner, do so. Boelte did, however, cut most processed carbs from his diet, so he could stay in the state of ketosis even when he ate, because he wasn't consuming any forms of glucose. This just proves that the combination of IF and a ketogenic diet is most beneficial even when not trying to lose weight.

Other

While the above health benefits are substantial and certainly the most popular, there are many more benefits. When your body is in the state of ketosis, many bodily functions are improved. This is due to a combination of resulting reactions that the body goes through after the metabolic switch. "IF regimens that induce the metabolic switch also induce the coordinated activation of signaling pathways that optimize physiological function, enhance performance and slow aging and disease processes" (Anton et al., 2018). So far, we've discussed some of these resulting reactions, such as autophagy and cellular repair, as well as the increase in energy production through mitochondria processes in the body's cells.

Another bodily function that is bettered is your brain function. When you're tired, you feel fuzzy, like you can't make decisions. This is because your brain function is the most important in the body, and it uses a lot of the energy your body produces. If it isn't getting enough power, it won't be able to run the entire body system, resulting in the fuzziness and confusion you experience when tired. When your brain is well fed, you won't feel confused because your cognitive function is stronger. When in ketosis, energy production is increased, allowing more energy for the brain to use. This results in not only better cognitive function, but also in better protection from neurodegenerative diseases like depression and Alzheimer's (Anton et al., 2018).

Other benefits of IF are improved blood pressure, reduced inflammation, better gut health, and of course, longevity. We've mentioned that hormone levels are better stabilized. Some of these include insulin and glucagon, as well as the appetite hormones ghrelin and leptin. Along with the processes of repair and rejuvenation of the entire body, these factors can contribute to the possible reversal of type 2 diabetes.

Chapter 3: A Fast Start — How it's Done

Now that you understand the processes your body goes through behind the curtains, as well as the different possible benefits of fasting, you can start to apply them to your own life. It will help you to understand the below timeframes and how each one is beneficial. Your personal results will naturally depend on your own situation, meaning, your dietary health, fitness level, mental health, and any medical issues. This is why you need to consider which timeline will work best for you, combined with whichever diet and exercise plan will benefit you personally. Hopefully, at this point, you are beginning to understand how longer fasts can help you lose more weight as well as let your body get to the process of repairing itself. But shorter fasts can be very beneficial as well; read on to find out how.

Fasting Schedules

We'll begin with the shorter fasting schedules and work our way up. Any fast that is 24 hours or under can be considered a short-term fast and can be done daily. Short-term fasts are beneficial because they regulate your insulin level by allowing it to stay low for a longer period of time and therefore decrease your risk for insulin resistance. As discussed, when you eat, your insulin level rises as it prepares to store excess energy. The longer that level stays up, the bigger your chances are for insulin resistance, which can cause a variety of health issues. As long as that level stays down, you're storing fewer and fewer fats as well as maintaining a healthy insulin balance.

16:8

The first number in the ratio is the fast length. This means that a person will fast for 16 hours and eat within the window of the remaining eight hours during the day. It can be shifted to whichever time frame suits you. For example, your eating window can be between 10 a.m. and 6 p.m. You might not even realize you're fasting on this regime because you could delay your breakfast and eat an earlier dinner. This way you can still eat three meals a day. If you don't eat breakfast, you can shift it to 12 p.m. to 8 p.m. Most find it easier to skip breakfast but eat lunch and dinner. However, there is talk about how eating breakfast is more beneficial because it can boost your energy for the day, although usually this is when people are doing workouts and need all the energy they can get.

18:6

This means you'll be fasting for 18 hours. Remember, this is when your body moves from the early fast state into the fasting state. This gives your body just enough time to start burning stored fats, but you won't be going into a state of ketosis. Your eating window is six hours. It's up to you when you want to use those six hours to eat according to your daily activity or your specific health goals. You can change it up and eat at different times of the day, as long as you keep track of your fasting period and get the best out of that.

20:4

Fast for 20 hours, eat during your four-hour window. You'll need to start considering your safety here as you need to last longer without food. If you feel dizzy or fatigued, eat again, but try to last a bit longer the next day. Your body should become used to it with time. However, if side effects persist, you should speak to your doctor before continuing. During your four-hour window, you need to remember to still eat as much as you would have before so that your body can still get all the nutrients and vitamins it needs. If your goal is weight loss, cut calories, not food.

24-hour, OMAD

One meal a day. Surprisingly, many people find this easy enough to do. Busy lifestyles mean less time to eat, much less prepare fresh and healthy meals. When put to the test, your busy schedule might distract you long enough to last until dinner time, when you should eat a large, balanced meal; large, not unhealthy, so that you can still get all the nutrients and vitamins that your body needs. As mentioned, it can be more beneficial to eat your big meal in the morning to get your energy up for the day, but most find it easier to skip breakfast.

>24-hour Schedules

Anything above a 24 hour fast is a long-term fast schedule. They're usually only done once or twice a week, depending on the length; however, fasts of 36 hours and up should be done less often. Any length of time above 18 hours will get you into the fasting state, so anything longer than 24 hours is even better. Considering that you would be entering the long-term fasting state after 48 hours, in terms of weight loss, the longer the better. However, it is more dangerous the longer you fast so be careful and please do talk to your health practitioner first. A popular time frame is 36 hours, as you can fast for a full 24 hour day and 12 hour night, and then eat again the next morning. This way, you'll be sleeping for technically two-thirds of your fast. The schedule is up to you, so you need to decide when you feel you'll need to replenish yourself again.

Intermittent Fasting Diet Plans According to Your Goals

For Losing Weight

While intermittent fasting is popular because it's a much less restrictive way to lose weight, you still need to help your body along. There won't be much of an improvement to your health if you're eating lots of carbohydrates and sugars. All that will happen is that all the extra sugar will be stored away quickly and efficiently and burning that stored fat off will become more and more difficult. Remember that if you want to see results, you'll need to eat fewer calories so that your stored fats keep decreasing instead of staying the same. If you continually top off your body with more stored fat after having fasted, you won't get very far in terms of weight loss. If you diet in a healthy way and avoid increasing your stored fat, eventually, you'll get to a point where your stored fat is decreasing every day. Always remember your health, though, cut calories, not food! You shouldn't be eating too much less than you normally do, as long as it's healthy food that you're filling up on.

So, what to eat then? Even though IF is said to have no rules, your diet should. Which dietary plan you choose is up to you, as long as it involves a measure of clean eating and tons of nutrient and vitamin intake. This won't only benefit your weight but your entire body as well, because those nutrients and vitamins are what help detox your body and keep all your organs running smoothly. If your organs are working well, your weight loss will become easier as your body assists you.

When I say that your diet should be clean, I mean you should avoid most processed and refined foods. Processed foods are anything that's been processed beyond their original fresh state. Examples are meats such as sausages, deli meats, or burgers and snacks such as potato chips or dried fruit.

Refined foods are mostly white grains such as white rice and pastas. There are many yummy alternatives, such as cauliflower rice or spinach pasta. Neither of these are new products, they've been around for a while, and many new products have been released since. Any plant-based grains will be great replacements. Adding them to your usual meals instead of carbohydrate-heavy starches will help you feel like you're still eating your normal meals.

Complex carbohydrates are good to eat as well, which are any grains not so heavily refined such as brown rice or anything whole wheat. These carbs, of course, should be excluded when following the ketogenic diet plan. If you are cutting carbohydrates from your diet, remember to eat fruits and vegetables high in fiber so your digestion still runs smoothly.

Meats and legumes (beans, lentils) are great for protein. Since you're fasting and your body is now taking energy from other parts of your body, protein within your muscles is one of them. So, increasing your protein intake could be a good idea to keep your muscle mass up and healthy so that your muscle can burn more calories.

Saving the best for last, fruits and vegetables are of course very important, especially now since your body is going to need all the nutrients it can get during your fasts. Try to balance out your veggie intake, as there are different families of vegetables, and they contain different vitamins, minerals and nutrients.

For a Longer, Healthier Life

While weight loss is definitely a major benefit, IF will change your health completely. As discussed in chapter two, a chain reaction of amazing processes begins within your body that detoxes cells and repairs and rejuvenates your entire body. There are many people who don't even want to lose weight but want to fix some kind of health issue or even just better their general health. Some health issues that IF can help with are high cholesterol, insulin resistance, cardiovascular health, diabetes, inflammation, and even depression. If you are looking to fix any of these issues, you should do a bit of specified research and find out just how IF can help you and which timelines and diet plans would be best for you. If you're looking to fix multiple issues and avoid any others, incorporating IF into your lifestyle is a great idea.

Many people say that they've noticed a change in their mood and overall focus since they started fasting regularly. If you suffer from anxiety or depression or even just constant bad moods, IF can help you gain more clarity and lift brain fog. Since your brain is getting more energy, it allows you to have better concentration and thought processing. Your body is getting more energy as well, so you don't feel sluggish or lazy. Your appetite hormones are being regulated so you don't feel as hungry. Combine all of these factors together and you have your reason for better moods. If you are getting a good night's sleep every night and keeping your stress low through meditation or whichever method you choose to use, the stress hormone, cortisol, will stay low and therefore keep you and your body calmer and more focused. With the addition of increase in healthy brain function you could even begin to overcome depression, on a chemical basis.

Please don't rely on IF completely if you suffer from depression, you will need to help your body along because fasting is only a supporting method to become healthier. The brain is supported by receiving more energy and therefore it can do its job more easily, by not only bettering moods but by preventing any neurodegenerative disease like depression, Alzheimer's or even Parkinson's (Anton et al., 2018). If you are susceptible to any of these diseases, if it runs in your family, you could prevent it or at least postpone it by incorporating IF into your lifestyle. This doesn't mean that you need to fast every day. If you can work some kind of fasting period in every month or a long fast every few months, you'll still benefit somewhat.

With your rise in energy levels (psychologically and physiologically), it won't be difficult for you to get up and get active more often, whether it's a full-blown workout or just a walk to the park. Activity isn't only for weight loss, we should all be active on a regular basis to keep our heart healthy, blood pressure low, and our muscles and bones strong. As mentioned, IF is a support method and you need to have a healthy lifestyle to reap benefits. If you are eating healthily, even with carbohydrates in your diet, you should be getting in enough nutrients and vitamins to support your body further. Every aspect of your diet or activity is a support mechanism, and the more support your body can get, the healthier you will be and the longer you will live. With the detoxification of your cells and increased cellular repair and growth, your body is equipped to prevent many diseases and illnesses.

Chapter 4: Outlast the Fast — Sustaining the Lifestyle

In the previous chapter, we discussed the lifelong benefits that you can gain from intermittent fasting. This won't happen if you only try it out every now and then. You'll have to fast regularly to have optimum health. Don't worry; it doesn't mean that you need to punish yourself in any way. Fasting isn't a punishment, merely a delay of gratification.

Once you've gotten the hang of it, you should find that you don't mind it too much. You can either use it as a daily routine, such as a 16:8 timeline where you can eat between 10 a.m. and 6 p.m., or you can use a longer fast every month, such as a 36-hour fast. You don't need to stick to the same timeline either. You can change it up or just fast when it's most convenient for you. Don't allow it to become a restriction in your life that stops you from enjoying a good night out or greasy family breakfast once in a while.

Some can get used to it very easily, and others will struggle. It all depends on various factors — your age and gender, your fitness level, even your susceptibility to addiction. Anything might be making it more difficult for you to get into the groove of fasting. The important thing to remember is that it shouldn't be difficult. If it isn't getting easier after a few tries, perhaps longer fasts just aren't for you, and you need to stick to a usual 12:12 regime. If you're constantly experiencing dizziness or fatigue, it would be a good idea to consult your doctor and make sure your blood pressure, cholesterol levels, as well as glucose and insulin levels are still at a healthy point. That aside, let's go over how you can outlast the fast and live a healthy life.

How to get Through a Fast

Hunger Management

Carbohydrates are a big hunger generator. If your body is used to a regular supply of carbohydrate-based glucose, it will crave it more and more. You could be one of the lucky ones and experience no hunger issues when fasting, but if you're used to a diet rich in carbs, the chances are that you'll get hungry. Another culprit of hunger pangs can be the frequency at which you're used to eating. If you've been eating small meals often or snacking in between meals, you'll probably struggle at first as well. But fear not, as intermittent fasting has the power to decrease those urges. When we discussed metabolism, we mentioned the hormones that control your appetite, namely ghrelin and leptin. When you fast regularly (or maintain a ketogenic diet as well as fasting) your body gets used to relying on stored fats for energy, so the appetite hormones stabilize, and you don't feel as hungry anymore. So, if you are experiencing severe hunger and it won't go away, you might need to consider cutting carbs from your diet or eating bigger meals less frequently throughout the day.

As for general hunger and merely pushing through the fast, there are some methods that can help distract you and your body. One example is to drink a glass of water anytime you feel like snacking. It will trick your body into thinking your stomach is full, and the cravings should subside somewhat. You could try drinking black tea or coffee with no sugar or enhancers added every time you feel the hunger rising. Caffeine is known to reduce appetite for a short while.

A more fun method of avoiding hunger is to sleep it off! If possible, try sleeping in later in the mornings and going to bed earlier at night. Not only will the sleep benefit you in various ways, but longer sleep equals longer fast. If you're fasting for a full day or few days, try taking naps to distract yourself, it's a healthy, cheap and no-fuss distraction! It's important to keep yourself busy and distracted. This means to do something that requires your full attention because this is a battle against your own mind. You won't starve during a fast (unless you're malnourished), so you just need to win the fight against your own body and mind. Practicing meditation and improving cognitive function through fasting will help you with this as you get more focused. You'll start to be able to control your own mind. Some people on forums about IF have mentioned that they feel they can now control their food, instead of their food controlling them (City-data Forum, n.d.). However, if mind over matter isn't your strong point, you should keep yourself busy with whatever you enjoy doing, whether it be sports or reading. Just keep that mind of yours occupied and you should outlast your fast.

The Metabolism Reset

The more scientific way to bust the hunger is to make that metabolic switch. It can only happen when your body is not relying on glucose for its energy supply. You'll need to avoid consuming any carbohydrates or sugars during your eating window in order to stay in the state of ketosis. This is how the ketogenic diet works and is why it is recommended to combine with intermittent fasting. They complement one another as fasting will help you reach a state of ketosis more quickly and easily, and your appetite is reduced when in ketosis state, assisting you during the fasts. When your body relies on ketones for energy, there is less stress on the cells because the energy derived from fats and amino acids is cleaner than that of sugar from carbohydrates. So, when your body is under less stress, not only will it run more smoothly, but it will have a calming effect on your mind. When you're hungry, you're stressed. It's a bodily reaction that puts you into an anxious state of need. If you can reduce your overall stress, hunger pangs shouldn't be as intense anymore.

All this worry about being hungry will become a non-issue as soon as your body becomes used to relying on ketones for energy. Ketosis is essentially a way for your body to preserve itself, so it stabilizes various hormones to avoid using too much energy on processes that aren't essential. This includes your appetite hormones, as mentioned in the previous section. Leptin is the hormone that suppresses your hunger. When you're in the state of ketosis, leptin is increased to help stabilize your system. If you can stay in this state or enter this state regularly, your hunger will decrease, and you won't feel the cravings as intensely. Those who have practiced resetting their metabolism have mostly said that they no longer feel hungry. When eating after a fast they feel full at a point and stop eating. Their bodies experience better control over appetite hormones and signal fullness to avoid overeating and storing more fat. Somehow, your body gets used to the healthier way of eating and helps you to regulate that.

How to Keep it up for Life

Fasting as a Health Regulator

Intermittent fasting isn't a diet plan, it's an eating pattern. Meaning it's not something you should do when you decide every few years you'd like to lose some weight, but rather something you incorporate into your lifestyle as a health regulator. We've gone over the many health benefits that IF can offer, that aren't just weight loss. IF can help regulate your health by keeping various hormone levels in check, increasing overall energy levels and brain function, and keeping you better protected against disease. If it still sounds daunting to you, don't stress. Many people don't fast all the time. They just fast from time to time to help their bodies remain detoxified and healthy. Every few months, if you can, give your body a good shock by fasting for 24-36 hours. Your body will make the metabolic switch within that time frame, rejuvenate body cells, and give your gut some time to stop digestion and get some rest.

I need to point out that not everyone can practice intermittent fasting. There are side effects that can impact anyone, namely dehydration, dizziness, headaches, and muscle pains. This eating method puts your body under an amount of stress. If it's more than you can handle, then it's not advised.

Persons who shouldn't play around with fasting are those who are more susceptible to addiction and eating disorders. This is a type of health issue that can run in the family so try to get to know your own health history and bodily traits before attempting any fasts. You won't be able to treat an eating disorder through fasting, it's too high risk for your mental health. Others who should avoid fasting are pregnant or breastfeeding women, as well as children. Anyone who's still growing needs that regular supply of food and energy. This relates to the malnourished. If a person is underweight or suffering from deficiencies, they will also need their regular supply of nutrients and energy.

Try Different Schedules

When incorporating IF into your lifestyle, you need to try various ways of fasting to find what works for you. If you struggle at first, it's okay, break your fast and eat. You can always try again. It's important that you don't deny yourself. Fasting should never feel like punishment. Considering what was said about eating disorders, you should never deny yourself to the point that you feel you need to binge eat and then feel guilty for doing so. Your meal after a fast should feel like a reward for being disciplined. That said, trying out different fasting schedules will help you to get a feel for the one that you find easiest. If you are an organized person who doesn't love change, you might find that keeping up the 16:8 fast as a daily routine is easiest and more satisfying for you. Whereas if you aren't a routine kind of person, doing a longer fast every now and then might work for you.

Life will intervene! As mentioned, you shouldn't deny yourself when life comes around; let yourself enjoy it. Go out with your friends late into the evening, eat a late dinner on date night, and have your early morning coffee with sugar and milk if you really need it to get through your day. Fasting will always be there for you tomorrow.

There are ways to use fasting when it's convenient for you. For example, you could follow an 18:6 schedule during the week, and then eat normally over weekends. Another example is to do a 36-hour fast once a month, when it's easy for you, whether that be during a busy workday or over a weekend. When Christmas comes around, ditch the fast for the month! There are always so many family gatherings and group dinners, you need to enjoy that time without worrying about fasting. Always remember that fasting is your friend, not your enemy. It's a support method and you won't die without it! If you are willing and able to fast for 24 hours after that big Christmas feast, go ahead.

Enjoy a Longer Life

If you can find a way to fast regularly, you'll enjoy a healthier and therefore longer life. The key word here is 'enjoy'. Use IF to your advantage, fit it in whenever you can. The whole reason for this method becoming popular is because it's a no-fuss method of weight and health control. It doesn't cost you a thing or force you to eat foods you actually hate. It's merely a scheduling matter and even that doesn't have to restrict you because you can stop fasting and start again whenever you'd like to. You won't lose any progress you've made by stopping the fast. Consider the fact that we all already fast while we sleep. Fasting is merely a continuation of that; put off breakfast for a few hours and you're intermittent fasting! Considering the significance of the health benefits and delaying a meal for a few hours should seem like a non-issue.

Once you've fasted a few times and have gotten used to a healthy lifestyle, you'll start to live your life with confidence that your health is covered. This isn't one of those cases where you don't see results and have to have blind faith. You will feel the results and you'll feel good. Your body will feel lighter because of energy increases and reduction of bloating. Your focus will improve and your moods along with it. If you've been living with hormone imbalances and the effects therefrom, you should notice the improvements. As the years pass, you won't age as quickly because your cells are being regularly refurbished. Did I forget to mention that you can tighten loose skin during the state of ketosis? Not only is this great for those losing weight but also for delaying the wrinkling process! As you grow older the aches and pains of aging won't affect you as easily because your body has become used to repairing itself and remaining at a calm state of stability. This stability is what will help you in the long run, because your body is under less stress. When your body is at a calm state and repairing itself constantly, your life span can be lengthened purely through a state of good health.

Conclusion: This is Your Fast Chance

Well, there you have it. Intermittent fasting in a relatively big nutshell. Hopefully, all of your questions have been answered through the scientific explanations and how to's. If you've been considering giving it a go, there is no time better than the present, or tomorrow morning, at least. Getting started is as easy as skipping breakfast.

Try IF out first by just extending the amount of time you aren't eating by an hour or two each day and see how it feels. When you feel it's manageable or easy enough, consider which schedule you'd like to try out first. By now you've probably already fasted for up to 18 hours so you can either carry on with an 18:6 schedule or challenge yourself with longer fasts. Shorter fasts will be easier to handle on an everyday basis, but if you struggle to keep up with the schedule, a longer fast once a week or once a month will do you well. It should actually be easier to keep up with a daily fasting schedule than a diet plan, as you don't have to eat specific foods at specific times but rather not eating at all at a specific time. The difficulty might lie in your hunger or various side effects. Once a week you can do a 24 or 36 hour fast, but anything longer you should only do once a month. Try to work it into your own schedule and find the best times to fast, when you're distracted or busy.

Remember that you need to be living a relatively healthy lifestyle before you can even consider fasting. Your body will need all the nutrients and vitamins it can get to keep your internal functions running smoothly during fasts. If you feel you aren't getting enough of a certain nutrient or vitamin, there are supplements you can consider taking to support your body's health. Supplements should not however be your first choice. Always try to get all the good stuff in through a healthy and balanced diet. Your best chance at having optimum health will be to combine a healthy diet with a good dose of regular activity and finally some regular fasting as well. You'll find that it will all become easier with time as you get used to it.

When you start to see results, use that sense of accomplishment to push further along and keep your healthy lifestyle up. You'll find that your mental health will become much more manageable with better moods and a more relaxed state of being. Remember to keep yourself hydrated with water and black coffee or tea, as your body needs to get used to the longer periods without an income of food. You'll feel the hunger at first, but it will subside. Drink more water if it helps you with the hunger, just not too much water as you could end up flushing out nutrients that your body will need now during its fasting state.

Take everything you've read here to heart and keep it there. All the science we've discussed should be general knowledge to everyone so that we can all live better and healthier lives. Fasting aside, you've read this book because you're concerned about keeping your body healthy and your life longer. There is no easy fix, until you learn that living a healthy lifestyle should be the only kind of lifestyle.

Processed foods will always be around but should be enjoyed in moderation. Once you feel that sense of pride when you've conquered a fasting regime and see the results, you'll start to understand how important it is, and it will seem easier to you. Anything will seem more difficult when you haven't tried it yet. Everything you've learned here isn't only applicable to intermittent fasting; all of it applies to our daily lives and our health as we age. If you learn anything from this book, let it be that fasting is a normal process of life that we all go through every night as we sleep. By learning how to control that process you can use it to your benefit and live a longer, healthier life.

If you enjoyed this book in anyway, an honest review is always appreciated!

References

Anton, S. D., Moehl, K., Donahoo, W. T., Marosi, K., Lee, S. A., Mainous, A. G., Leeuwenburgh, C., & Mattson, M. P. (2018). Flipping the Metabolic Switch: Understanding and Applying the Health Benefits of Fasting. *Obesity (Silver Spring, Md.)*, 26(2), 254–268. https://doi.org/10.1002/oby.22065

Boelte, K. (2017, May 10). *What I Learned from a Year of Intermittent Fasting*. Outside Online. https://www.outsideonline.com/2181151/what-i-learned-year-intermittent-fasting

Britannica, T. E. of E. (2021). Fasting. In *Encyclopædia Britannica*. https://www.britannica.com/topic/fasting

City-data Forum. (n.d.). *Intermittent Fasting, what results have you seen? (overweight, systems, doctors) - Diet and Weight Loss - Weight management - City-Data Forum*. Www.city-Data.com. Retrieved April 24, 2021, from http://www.city-data.com/forum/diet-weight-loss/3069803-intermittent-fasting-what-results-have-you.html

Gunnars, K. (2016, August 16). *10 Evidence-Based Health Benefits of Intermittent Fasting*. Healthline. https://www.healthline.com/nutrition/10-health-benefits-of-intermittent-fasting#TOC_TITLE_HDR_7

Langness, D. (2019, March 3). *When and Why Did Humans Start Fasting?* Bahaiteachings.org/. https://bahaiteachings.org/when-why-did-humans-start-fasting/

Pannell, N. (2018, August 27). *10 things you've heard about intermittent fasting that aren't true*. Insider. https://www.insider.com/intermittent-fasting-myths-2018-8#myth-fasting-will-slow-your-metabolism-down-2

Puckett, S. (2020, January 20). *Fasting for Your Health: What You Need to Know*. Boulder Medical Center. https://www.bouldermedicalcenter.com/6703-2/#:~:text=Essentially%2C%20fasting%20cleanses%20our%20body

Shanks, K. (2019, August 16). *How to Boost Energy with Ketosis and Intermittent Fasting*. Karyn Shanks MD. https://www.karynshanksmd.com/2019/08/16/energy-ketosis-intermittent-fasting/

www.ingramcontent.com/pod-product-compliance
Lightning Source LLC
Chambersburg PA
CBHW032100040426
42336CB00039B/509